Porn is a Question of Cosmological Significance

From the "Best Works" series

CJS Hayward

CJS Hayward Publications, Spotsylvania

To St. Mary of Egypt—
One of the greatest ascetics in history,
A first class friend of those seeking chastity,
And a shining example of what second virginity can look like!

Table of Contents

Introduction

There are many issues and difficulties surrounding technology, but among these issues, porn is simply not one issue among others. It used to be the number one confessed sin among young men, and now it is the most confessed sin, period. And this is among people who know it to be wrong.

St. John Chrysostom perennially warned about the obscene theaters in which "the shared nature of women is insulted." Now almost all of us, and on all continents, carry a porn delivery system in our pocket. Porn is a pack of cigarettes for the soul. Porn is the disenchantment of the entire universe, a festering-ground for cruelty and anger, the destruction of pleasure, a trapdoor of impotence, the gateway drug to being jailed for rape. But you may have more freedom than you realize, and part of it has to do with how we tend to view porn.

This is a book intended to enable the reader to never look the same way at porn ever again.

To those who have never used porn and are faithful / chaste—enjoy the book, and keep being awesome!

To fellow strugglers with sexual sin—*this book is written for you!*

This collection comprises four works:

1. " 'Porn?' is a Question of Cosmological Significance" is intended to look at what is really at stake in the question of porn, and that is really quite a lot.

2. "A Pet Owner's Rules" is a homily that tackles several prominent sins. And really, porn is not the only sin out there, but it is the one most frequently brought to confession. This homily is meant to help you resist all sin.

3. "The Magic Stone" is written because in technological addiction, even without porn being in the picture, spiritual factors make it seem like there is nothing else to do besides plugging in. This mentions a hundred and more things that you can do that do not include porn.

4. "Fire in the Hole" is named after the military command for when an explosion in a confined space is imminent. The hero is a professor who is able to say and back up, "Do you like porn? I have something better to offer you."

Enjoy!

(P.S. If you'd like to read the story behind the saint to whom this work is dedicated, the life of St. Mary of Egypt at tinyurl.com/st-mary-of-egypt is well worth reading or re-reading!)

Porn is a Question of Cosmological Significance

Another question of cosmological significance

In my second master's thesis, "AI as an Arena for Magical Thinking Among Skeptics,"[1] I have a section, "Intellect, Principles, and Cosmology," in which I wrote:

> Why do I speak of the 'artificial intelligence cosmology'? Surely one can have a long debate about artificial intelligence without adding cosmology to the discussion. This is true, but it is true because cosmology has become invisible, part of the assumed backdrop of

discussion. In America, one cultural assumption is that 'culture' and 'customs' are for faroff and exotic people, not for 'us'—'we' are just being human. It doesn't occur to most Americans to think of eating Turkey on Thanksgiving Day or removing one's hat inside a building as customs, because 'custom' is a concept that only applies to exotic people. I suggest that Maximus Confessor has an interesting cosmology, not because he's exotic, but because he's human.

Artificial intelligence proponents and (most) critics do not differ on cosmology, but because that is because it is an important assumption which is not questioned even by most people who deny the possibility of artificial intelligence. Searle may disagree with Fodor about what is implied by a materialist cosmology, but not whether one should accept materialism. I suggest that some artificial intelligence critics miss the most interesting critiques of artificial intelligence because they share that project's cosmology. If AI is based on a cosmological error, then no amount of fine-tuning within the system will rectify the error. We need to consider cosmology if we are to have any hope of correcting an error that basic. (Bad metaphysics does not create good physics.) I will describe Maximus Confessor's cosmology in this section, not because he has cosmology and AI doesn't, but because his cosmology seems to suggest a correction to the artificial intelligence cosmology.

At the base of Maximus's cosmology is God. God holds the Principles in his heart, and they share something of his reality. Concrete beings (including us) are created through the Principles, and we share something of their reality and of God. The Principles are a more concrete realisation of God, and we are a more concrete realisation of the Principles. Thought (nohsis) means beholding God and the Principles (logoi) through the eye of the intellect. Thinking of a tree means connecting with something that is more tree-like than the tree itself.

It may be easier to see what the important Principles in Maximus Confessor's cosmology if we see how they are being dismantled today. Without saying that Church Fathers simply grafted in Platonism, I believe it safe to say that Plato resembled some of Church doctrine, and at any rate Plato's one finger pointing up to God offers a closer approximation to Christianity than Aristotle's fingers pointing down. I would suggest further that looking at Plato can suggest how Christianity differs from Aristotelianism's materialistic tendencies, tendencies that are still unfolding today. Edelman describes the assumptions

accompanying Darwin's evolution as the
'death blow' to the essentialism, the doctrine
that there are fixed kinds of things, as taught
by Plato and other idealists.[46] Edelman
seems not to appreciate why so many
biologists assent to punctuated equilibrium.
[47] However, if we assume that there is solid
evidence establishing that all life gradually
evolved from a common ancestor, then this
remark is both apropos and perceptive.

The cosmology shared by the artificial intelligence
movement and its mainstream critics within the academy is
a standard scientific cosmology in which, in particular, the
royal race of mankind is in fact an unintended by-product of
mindless forces that did not in any sense have the human
race in desire or mind. The debate between John Searle and
"strong AI" proponents is not about whether this whole
cosmology holds. It is not about whether a part of this
cosmology holds. It is rather that given the complete truth
of the cosmology, there is a difference about whether it
implies that computers can replicate intelligence such as the
royal race of men possess."

Regarding that cosmology, I would quote "The
Commentary:"[2]

Martin stepped into his house and decided to
have no more distractions. He wanted to begin
reading commentary, now. He opened the book
on the table and sat erect in his chair:

Genesis

1:1 In the beginning God
created the heavens and the
earth.
1:2 The earth was without
form and void, and
darkness was upon the face
of the deep; and the Spirit
of God was moving over the
face of the waters.
1:3 And God said, "Let
there be light"; and there
was light.

The reader is now thinking about
evolution. He is wondering whether
Genesis 1 is right, and evolution is
simply wrong, or whether evolution is
right, and Genesis 1 is a myth that may
be inspiring enough but does not
actually tell how the world was
created.

All of this is because of a culture
phenomenally influenced by scientism
and science. The theory of evolution is
an attempt to map out, in terms
appropriate to scientific dialogue, just
what organisms occurred, when, and
what mechanism led there to be new
kinds of organisms that did not exist

before. Therefore, nearly all
Evangelicals assumed, Genesis 1 must
be the Christian substitute for
evolution. Its purpose must also be to
map out what occurred when, to
provide the same sort of mechanism.
In short, if Genesis 1 is true, then it
must be trying to answer the same
question as evolution, only answering
it differently.

Darwinian evolution is not a true
answer to the question, "Why is there
life as we know it?" Evolution is on
philosophical grounds not a true
answer to that question, because it is
not an answer to that question at all.
Even if it is true, evolution is only an
answer to the question, "How is there
life as we know it?" If someone asks,
"Why is there this life that we see?"
and someone answers, "Evolution," it
is like someone saying, "Why is the
kitchen light on?" and someone else
answering, "Because the switch is in
the on position, thereby closing the
electrical circuit and allowing current
to flow through the bulb, which grows
hot and produces light."

Where the reader only sees one
question, an ancient reader saw at

least two other questions that are
invisible to the present reader. As well
as the question of "How?" that
evolution addresses, there is the
question of "Why?" and "What
function does it serve?" These two
questions are very important, and are
not even considered when people are
only trying to work out the
antagonism between creationism and
evolutionism.

Martin took a deep breath. Was the text
advocating a six-day creationism? That was hard
to tell. He felt uncomfortable, in a much deeper
way than if Bible-thumpers were preaching to
him that evolutionists would burn in Hell.

What is the cosmological issue? I quote "Within the
Steel Orb:"[3]

Art said, "But our scientists are making
progress. Your advanced world has artificial
intelligence, right?"

Oinos said, "Why on earth would we be able to
do that? Why would that even be a goal?"

"You have computers, right?"

3   cjshayward.com/steel

"Yes, indeed; the table that I used to call up a scientific calculator works on the same principle as your world's computers. I could almost say that inventing a new kind of computer is a rite of passage among serious inventors, or at least that's the closest term your world would have."

"And your computer science is pretty advanced, right? Much more advanced than ours?"

"We know things that the trajectory of computer science in your world will never reach because it is not pointed in the right direction." Oinos tapped the wall and arcs of pale blue light spun out.

"Then you should be well beyond the point of making artificial intelligence."

"Why on a million, million worlds should we ever be able to do that? Or even think that is something we could accomplish?"

"Well, if I can be obvious, the brain is a computer, and the mind is its software."

"Is it?"

"What else could the mind be?"

"What else could the mind be? What about an altar at which to worship? A workshop? A bridge between Heaven and earth, a meeting place where eternity meets time? A treasury in which to gather riches? A spark of divine fire? A line in a strong grid? A river, ever flowing, ever full? A tree reaching to Heaven while its roots grasp the earth? A mountain made immovable for the greatest storm? A home in which to live and a ship by which to sail? A constellation of stars? A temple that sanctifies the earth? A force to draw things in? A captain directing a starship or a voyager who can travel without? A diamond forged over aeons from of old? A perpetual motion machine that is simply impossible but functions anyway? A faithful manuscript by which an ancient book passes on? A showcase of holy icons? A mirror, clear or clouded? A wind which can never be pinned down? A haunting moment? A home with which to welcome others, and a mouth with which to kiss? A strand of a web? An acrobat balancing for his whole life long on a slender crystalline prism between two chasms? A protecting veil and a concealing mist? An eye to glimpse the uncreated Light as the world moves on its way? A rift yawning into the depths of the earth? A kairometer, both primeval and young? A—"

"All right, all right! I get the idea, and that's some pretty lovely poetry. (What's a kairometer?) These are all very beautiful metaphors for the mind, but I am interested in what the mind is literally."

"Then it might interest you to hear that your world's computer is also a metaphor for the mind. A good and poetic metaphor, perhaps, but a metaphor, and one that is better to balance with other complementary metaphors. It is the habit of some in your world to understand the human mind through the metaphor of the latest technology for you to be infatuated with. Today, the mind is a computer, or something like that. Before you had the computer, 'You're just wired that way' because the brain or the mind or whatever is a wired-up telephone exchange, the telephone exchange being your previous object of technological infatuation, before the computer. Admittedly, 'the mind is a computer' is an attractive metaphor. But there is some fundamental confusion in taking that metaphor literally and assuming that, since the mind is a computer, all you have to do is make some more progress with technology and research and you can give a computer an intelligent mind."

The setting is science fiction and the litany of metaphors is meant to be literally true as a litany of metaphors in which "The brain is a computer" fits as one metaphor among others and not the one metaphor that is in fact literal truth.

What other kinds of cosmological questions are there?

There is a standard block of dummy text used in print design and by designers on the web. It is called "lorem ipsum," and it has been traced as a lightly mangled version of "De Finis Bonorum et Malorem," section 1.10.32, which happens to be an original text of (tr. 1914 H Rackam):[4]

But I must explain to you how all this mistaken idea of denouncing pleasure and praising pain was born and I will give you a complete account of the system, and expound the actual teachings of the great explorer of the truth, the master-builder of human happiness. No one rejects, dislikes, or avoids pleasure itself, because it is pleasure, but because those who do not know how to pursue pleasure rationally encounter consequences that are extremely painful. Nor again is there anyone who loves or pursues or desires to obtain pain of itself, because it is pain, but because occasionally circumstances occur in which toil and pain can procure him some great pleasure. To take a trivial example, which of us ever undertakes laborious physical exercise, except to obtain some advantage from it? But who has any right to find fault with a man who chooses to enjoy a

pleasure that has no annoying consequences,
or one who avoids a pain that produces no
resultant pleasure?

St. Paul quotes a proverb in the same vein as, "Let us
eat and drink, for to morrow we die." This is mentioned in
relation to the greatest chapter in the Pauline letters about
the resurrection which is pre-emiment among Christian
hopes. Hedonism, as in the *carpe diem* that leads to
suicide in *Dead Poets Society*, is not a joyful philosophy at
all. It is a philosophy that says we might as well eat, drink,
and be merry, because there is no greater good to be had
than pleasure in this rapidly vanishing life.
To this I say, "There are more things in Heaven and
earth than are dreamed of in this philosophy."

A question on par with cosmology, worldview, and the Way in which we walk

If one accepts a worldview under which hedonism is
a straightforward available option, including the moralistic
therapeutic deism that Rob Dreher says is "mostly about
improving one's self-esteem and subjective happiness and
getting along well with others" in *The Benedict Option*, then
condemning porn is an uprooted plant that is placed in dry
sand and has no way to draw real water. It will likely be
short-lived. At least for the person who is tempted to use
porn, the "thou shalt not" is an uprooted plant at a loss for
sustenance to draw on. Now feminism may be able to
scathingly condemn porn and say in a feminist dictionary,

"Pornography is the theory. Rape is the practice." However, the initial pleasure that porn seems like it will offer is strong, and a rootless "Thou shalt not" has a very uphill battle to wage.

But the "Thou shalt not" does not need to be rootless. It is not rootless under Orthodox cosmology, worldview, or Way. And I say this even if I use the term "worldview" advisedly because the semiotic frame of "worldview" is something one has to pioneeringly construct and not something that has already been established, needs our curation and not pioneering from scratch, and has to do with an Athonite elder saying, "It's not 'Take what the previous version has kept unchanged, and pass it on unchanged to the next generation;' it's 'Take what the previous generation worked on, work on it, and pass it on to the next generation to work on.'" The worldview *aspect* of Orthodox Tradition is not the sort of thing one should *construct*; it is something to *conserve, adapt,* and *keep custody of,* even or especially if "to conserve is to change."

The cosmic picture we live in is of a world more wondrous than George MacDonald's fairy-land and fairy tales. It is of an entire cosmos that does not exist apart from a Creator (Aristotelianism said matter had always existed and was merely given form by God), nor for instance as in Babylonian mythology did a warrior-god tear the dragon Tiamat and make one part the earth and the other part the sky, nor one of mindless forces playing out as in the gospel according to modern science, but an entire world created with beauty and purpose, an entire world and everything in it the creation of a loving and infinitely wise God, embedded in the story beyond all other stories, a God who is the best of all possible Gods and exercises towards us the best of all possible Providences. It is a world in which this present life is of unspeakably great importance, during which we make an eternal choice between being everlasting splendors shining the uncreated Light, and horrors beyond being a nightmare. It is as I wrote before being Orthodox, in one not-so-great novella,

> I would like to tell you a story. I prayed, and hesitated now — Lord, I pray, bind me from saying anything that would harm these little ones, bind the power of the Evil One, and keep me in your heart. But I'll tell the story, with a warning that I don't agree with all of it. When I told it to one young man, he asked me, 'So, do you really believe that God created man just to prove a point?' I stepped back and said, 'No. I don't believe that. That's not why I told the story at all; it's just that I don't know how to tell the story without it looking that way.' So I ask you to excuse my weakness, and I pray that you will see what in this story I mean to tell: God's power and wisdom as manifest in his redemption.
>
> "In the very beginning, before God created the heavens and the earth, he created angels, stars of light to shine in the light of glory. He created one star higher and holier than any of the others, and named him Lucifer, the Light-Bearer.

"Lucifer saw his own wisdom, majesty and glory, and told God, 'I want you to give me my rightful place, as head of you as well as head of the angels. I am wiser than you.'

"God could have zapped Lucifer then and there, and that would have established his power. But not his wisdom. So God decided on something very different.

"'Very well, then,' God said, 'Prove it. I'll unfold my plan, and you'll unfold yours.'

"The great Dragon shouted in rebellion, and swept the sky with his tail, and flung down a third of the stars, and a third of the stars chose to become dragons, vipers, worms.

"Then God created Heaven and earth; he set the stars, in their courses, and created glory after glory after glory: no two blades of grass alike, thousands upon thousands of species of beetles, and as the crowning glory man, created godlike in his image, pure, holy, spotless.

"Then the Dragon appeared in the form of a serpent, and beguiled the woman, and the woman pulled the man down with her. The whole creation became accursed, and began to rot, with poison seeping in a wound.

"'Well, then,' the Dragon said, 'Who is wiser now?' And God wept.

"Then God pointed to one person and said, 'You see that man?'

"'Yes,' the Devil said.

"'Hey, there!' God said to the man. 'You in the desert. Build a huge boat.'

"And the man did. When the wind and rain came, the man and his household were saved.

"Then the Devil walked on the earth, and said, 'I see not one who is righteous,' and God said, 'Have you considered my servant Job?' And Job, bewildered, saw his children and his property taken away, and then his health — and cried in agony, cursing the day of his birth, but refusing to curse God like the Serpent said he would. In the midst of his misery, Job said, 'I know that my redeemer liveth, and in my flesh I shall see God. Though he slay me, yet shall I praise him.'

"The story unfolded, and God sent a prophet to give his people Law. When they strayed, he sent prophets, never tiring of loving them. Finally, in the fullness of time, he sent his Son, to become a man.

"This man was a stranger in a strange land, and passed through the world like a flame. The Serpent spoke beguiling words into the ear of one of his disciples, and he was betrayed, and nailed to a piece of wood, and left to die. And darkness reigned.

"'Surely you will acknowledge,' said the Serpent, 'that I am wiser?'

"God raised his Son from the dead, in a new and incorruptible life, surging with power. And the Devil trembled with fear.

"His Spirit filled those who were his Son's disciples, and they burst forth with new life. The Serpent tried everything to stop them — even making some of the people God had called to persecute them. God was not discouraged; he called one of the persecutors to join in the new life." The preacher took off his glasses, and said, "I'd like to read to you now from one of the letters written by that persecutor:

"'Although I am less than the least of all God's people, this grace was given me: to preach to the Gentiles the unsearchable riches of Christ, and to make plain to everyone the administration of this mystery, which for ages past was kept hidden in God, who created all things. His intent was that now, through the church, the manifold wisdom of God should be made known to the rulers and authorities in the heavenly realms, according to his eternal purpose which he accomplished in Christ Jesus our Lord.'

"The Church — I mean you and me, not just people who wear a white collar — stands as a family for Christ, his brother and sister and mother, as children for God the Father, as God's *magnum opus*, as a servant to the world, as a witness to the world, as a mother and family to those who believe, and lastly as a warrior against Satan. This is the secret God has concealed in his bosom, and his many-sided wisdom is displaying so that all of the angels and even all of the demons, Satan himself, can look and see the wisdom of God's plan.

"Christ came once; he will come again, and then every knee shall bow. Then the redeemed shall stand holy, spotless, pure, and perfect, gods and goddesses, sons and daughters of God, to enter into his eternal paradise. Then the Dragon will look and see beyond any question or doubt that God's plan is wiser. Then, and *only* then, will Satan and all his minions be cast into the lake of eternal fire.

The Orthodox word and narrative is one that places us in a tremendously important world. For one detail,

"Examples of the kiss as a means of making and breaking enchantments have been found in the fairy tales of virtually every culture in the Western world." Christians share a holy kiss that is the only act the Bible calls holy, and the Sacrament of Sacraments is itself illuminated as kiss: as Orthodox pray before communion, "Neither will I give Thee a kiss as did Judas." The entire universe has order: the entire universe has meaning: the entire universe is called to dance the great dance.

And in that world, one of the richest ecclesiological passages in the Bible reads:

> ...submitting yourselves one to another in the fear of God.

> Wives, unto your own husbands, as unto the Lord. For the husband is the head of the wife, even as Christ is the Head of the Church: and he is the Saviour of the body. Therefore as the Church is subject unto Christ, so let the wives be to their own husbands in every thing. Husbands, love your wives, even as Christ also loved the Church, and gave Himself up for her; that He might sanctify and cleanse her with the washing of water by the word, that He might present her to Himself a glorious Church, not having spot, or wrinkle, or any such thing; but that it should be holy and without blemish. So ought men to love their wives as their own bodies. He that loveth his wife loveth himself. For no man ever yet hated his own flesh; but nourisheth and cherisheth

it, even as the Lord the Church: for we are
members of His body, of His flesh, and of His
bones. "For this cause shall a man leave his
father and mother, and shall be joined unto
his wife, and they two shall be one flesh." This
is a great mystery: but I speak concerning
Christ and the Church. Let every one of you in
particular so love his wife even as himself; and
the wife see that she reverence her husband.

The passage is chokingly politically incorrect even if
it places a much heavier burden on husbands than on wives,
but Christ and the Church find a signally important icon in
the sacrament of marriage between one man and one
woman, or if I may underscore the point, the marriage
between one lord and one wife. And if this seems
demeaning, I would invite you to watch Disney's classic
cartoon of Beauty and the Beast. Every little girl wants to
marry a Prince; and the natural desire of woman is to marry
a lord, however much we try to legislate it away.

Furthermore, the truth of headship extends far
beyond political incorrectness about one lord and one wife.
It extends to:

Today I'm going to talk about head and body
(headship). And I say "headship" with
hesitation, because in today's world asserting
"headship" means, "defending traditional
gender roles against feminism." And that
maybe important, but I want to talk about
something larger, something that will be
missed if "headship" means nothing more

than "one position in the feminist controversy."

One speaker didn't like people entering Church and saying, "It's so good to enter the Lord's presence." He said, "Where were you all week? How did you escape the Lord's presence?" And whatever Church is, it is absolutely not entering the one place where God is present. At least, it's not stepping out of some imaginary place where God simply can't be found.

But if we are always in the Lord's presence, that doesn't mean that Church isn't special. It is special, and it is the head of living in God's presence for all of our lives. Our time in Church is an example of headship. Worshipping God in Church is the head of a life of worship, and it is the head of a body.

There is something special about our time in Church. But the way we live our lives, our "body" of time spent, manifests that glory in a different way. Christ didn't say that people will know we are his disciples by our "official" worship, however much God's blessing may rest on it. Christ said instead that all people will know we are his disciples by this, that we love one another. That isn't primarily in Church. That's in our day to day lives. If our time in Church crystallizes a life of worship,

our love for one another is to manifest it. And
that is the place of the body.

The relationship between head and body is the
relationship between corporate worship and
our lives as a whole. The body manifests the
glory of the head. In my head I can decide to
walk to a friend's house. But the head needs
the body and the body needs the head, and I
can only go to a friend's house if my head's
decision to visit a friend's house is lived out in
my body. "The head cannot say to the feet, 'I
have no need of you.'"

The Father is the head of the Son. "No man
can see God and live." God the Father is
utterly beyond us; he transcends anything we
could know; he is pure glory. If we were to
have direct contact with him, we would be
destroyed. And yet the Son is equal to the
Father; the Son is just as far beyond this
Creation, but there is a difference. The Son is
the bridge between God and man, and God
and his Creation. God the Father created the
world through the Son, and the Son is just as
glorious as the Father, but the Son can touch
us without destroying us. The Father displays
himself through the Son. The Father's love
came to earth through the Son. The Father's
wish that we may be made divine is possible
precisely because the Son became man. And
finally we can know the Father through the

Son. If you have seen the Son, you have seen the Father.

We read in the New Testament that Christ is the head of man, that Christ is the head of all authority, that Christ is the head of the Church, and that Christ is the head of the whole Creation. If we think, with people today, that to have any authority over us, any head, is degrading, then we have to resent a lot more than a husband's headship to his wife. But that's not the only option. When Christ is the head of the cosmos, there is more than authority going on, even if we have a negative view of authority. Our Orthodox understanding that the Son of God became a man that men might become the sons of God, that the divine became human that the human might become divine, expresses what the headship of Christ means. Christ is the head, and that means that the Church is drawn up in his divinity. If we are the body of Christ the head, that doesn't mean we're just under his authority. It means that we are a part of him and share in his divinity. The teaching that we share in his divinity is very tightly connected to the teaching of "recapitulation", or "re-heading," where Christ being the head of the Church, and our sharing in Christ's divinity, are two sides of the same coin. Christ is the head, and we, the body, make Christ manifest to the world. Some people may not know

Christ except what they see in us. We cannot have Christ as our head without being a manifestation of his glory, and if Christ is the head of the Creation and Christ is the head of the Church, that means that when we worship, inside this building and in our daily lives, we are leading the whole visible Creation in turning to God in glory, and living the life of Heaven here on earth.

Christ is the head of the whole Creation, not just the Church. Christ isn't just concerned with his people, but the whole created world. By him and through him all things were created. Icons, which reflect the full implications Christ's headship over his Creation, exist precisely because Christ is the head of the whole Creation. We use a censer, a building, icons, water, flowers, and other aspects of our matter-embracing religion as representatives of the whole material Creation over which Christ is head. Christ doesn't tell us to be spiritual as spirits who are unfortunately trapped in matter; far from it, we are the crowning jewel of the material Creation, and Christ's headship glorifies the whole Creation and makes it foundational to how we are saved. The universe is a symbol that manifests the glory of its head, Christ.

One example of headship that is immediate to me, although I don't know how immediate it is to the rest of you, is artistic creation. I create, write, and program, and in a very real sense I am at my fullest when I create. When I create, at first there is a hazy idea that I don't understand very well. Then I listen to it, and begin struggling with it, trying to understand my creation, and even if I am wrestling with it, I am wrestling less to dominate it than to get myself out of its way so I can help bring it into being. If in one sense I wrestle with it, in another sense I am wrestling with myself to let my creation be what it should be. If I were to simply dominate my creation, I would crush it, breaking its spirit. My best creations are those which I serve, where I use my headship to give my creations freedom and cooperate with them so that they are greater than if I did not give my creations room to breathe. My best work comes, not when I decide, "I am going to create," but when I cooperate with a creation, love it, serve it, and help it to become real, the creation becomes a share of my spirit.

A great many writers could say that, and I don't think this is something that is only found in writing, but how something far more general plays out. All of us are called to exercise headship over our work. In a family, the father is the head of the household and the mother is the heart of the household. The mother's headship over work in the home provides ten thousand touches that make a house a home. A mother's headship over the home is as much human headship over one's work as my headship over my creations and writing. What I do when I create is love my creation, serve it, develop it, work with God and with my creation to help it be real. If I'm not mistaken, when a woman makes a house into a real home, she loves it, serves it, develops it, and works with God and what she has to make it real. When a woman makes a house into a warm and inviting home, *that's headship*.

What is the relationship between women and the home? In societies where people have best been able to honor what the Bible says about men's and women's roles, there is a strong association between women and the home. The home, in those societies, was the main focus of business, charity work, and education, besides the much narrower role played by a home today. To say that women were mainly in the home is to say that they held an important place in one of society's important institutions, an institution that was the chief home of business, education, hospitality, and what would today be insurance, and held many responsibilities that are denied to housewives today. The isolation felt by many housewives today was much less an issue because women worked together with other women; like men, they worked in adult company. I believe there should be an association between women and the home, and I believe the home should be respected and influential. And, for that matter, I believe that both men and women are sold short with the options they have today. But instead of going too deep into that sort of question, important as it may be, I would like to look at what headship means.

The sanctuary is the head of the nave. Part of what that means is that there is something richer than either if there were just an sanctuary or just a nave. But we'll miss something fundamental if we only say that the sanctuary is more glorious to the nave. They are connected and part of the same body. They are part of the same organism, and the sanctuary manifests the glory of the sanctuary. There is also a head-body relation between the saint and the icon. Or between the reality a symbol represents, and a symbol. Or between Heaven and earth. Bringing Heaven down to earth is a right ordering of this world. Heaven isn't just something that happens after death after we serve God by suffering in this world. "Eye has not seen, ear has not heard, nor has any heart imagined what God has prepared for those who love him," but God wants to work Heaven in our lives, beginning here and now. If we are bringing Heaven down to earth, we are realizing God's design that Heaven be the head of earth, in the fullness of what headship means.

What about husbands and wives? There's something that we'll miss today if we just expect wives to submit to their husbands, even if we recognized that that's tied to an even more difficult assignment for husbands, loving their wives on the model of Christ giving up his own life for the Church. And we need to be countercultural, but there's something we'll miss if we just react to the currents in society that make this unattractive. Quite a few heresies got their start in reactions against older heresies; it is spiritually dangerous to simply react against errors, and if feminism might have problems, simply reacting to feminism is likely to have problems. Wives should submit to their husbands, and husbands should love their wives with a costly love, but there's more.

It bothers me when conservatives say, "I want to turn the clock back... all the way back... *to 1954!*" If we're just reacting against some feminists when they say women should be strong and independent, and have no further reference point, we're likely to defend a femininity that says that women are weak and passive. What's wrong with that? For starters, it's not Biblical.

If you want to know God's version of
femininity, read the conclusion of Proverbs.
The opening of this conclusion is often
translated, "Who can find a good wife?" That's
too weak. It is better translated as, "Who can
find a wife of **valor**," with "valor" being a
word that could be used of a mighty soldier.
She is strong—physically *strong*. The text
explicitly mentions her powerful arms. She is
active in commerce and charity. There are
important differences between this and the
feminist picture, but if we are defending an
un-Biblical ideal for womanhood, some
delicate thing that can't do anything and is
always in a swoon, then our reaction against
feminism isn't going to put us in a much better
spot.

And men should be men, but that doesn't
mean that men should be rugged individuals
who say, "I am the master of my fate: I am the
captain of my soul!" That is as wrong as saying
that Biblical femininity is weak and passive.
Perhaps men should be rugged, but to be a
man is to be under authority. Trying to be the
captain of your soul is spiritually toxic, and
perhaps blasphemous. There is one person
who can say, "I am the captain of my soul,"
and it isn't Christ. Not even Christ can say
that, but only God the Father. Christ's glory
was to be the Son of God, so that the Father
was the captain of his soul, and he did the

Father's work. Even Christ was under the headship of the Father, and if you read what John says about the Father and the Son, the fact that Christ was under headship, under authority, is part of his dignity and his own authority. To be a man is, if things are going well, to be a contributing member of a community, and in submission to its authority. Individualism is a severe distortion of masculinity; it may not be feminine, but it is hardly characteristic of healthy masculinity. There are a lot of false and destructive pictures of what a man should be, as well as what a woman should be.

If simply reacting against feminism is a way to miss what it means to be a man and what it means to be a woman, it is also a way to miss something more, to miss a broader glory. This something more is foundational to the structure of reality; it is a resonance not only with God's Creation, but within the nature of God and how the Father's glory is shown through the Son. This something more is in continuity with God's headship to Christ, Christ's headship to the Church, Christ's headship to the cosmos, Heaven's headship to earth, the sanctuary's headship to the nave, the spiritual world's headship to the physical world, the soul's headship to the body, contemplation's headship to action, and other manifestations of a headship relation. On the Sunday of Orthodoxy, we proclaim:

> ...Thus we declare, thus we assert, thus we preach Christ our true God, and honor as Saints in words, in writings, in thoughts, in sacrifices, in churches, in Holy Icons; on the one hand worshipping and reverencing Christ as God and Lord, and on the other hand honoring as true servants of the same Lord of all and accordingly offering them veneration... This is the Faith of the Apostles, this is the Faith of the Fathers, this is the Faith of the Orthodox, this is the Faith which has established the Universe.

What does this have to do with heads and bodies? The word "icon" itself means a body, and its role is to manifest the glory of the saints, as the saints are to manifest the glory of God.

We don't have a choice about whether we will live in a universe with headship, but we do have a choice whether to work with the grain or against it, work with it to our profit or fight it to our detriment. Let's make headship part of how we rejoice in God and his Creation.

And where is porn in all this?

Pornography is like trying to seek warmth, not by putting a sweater, but by lighting part of your house on fire.

It does deliver impressive warmth quickly, but this is bitterly fleeting: if Proverbs says that the adulterous woman is in the beginning as sweet as honey and in the end as bitter as gall and as sharp as a double edged sword, then the adulterous woman chastises with whips while porn chastises with scorpions.

Porn is like a dog licking a saw: it likes the taste but the taste is the taste of its own woundedness. Porn is anonymous sex. Masturbating after porn, the masturbatory act, the act that porn viewing leads into, is an ultimate exploitation of the model(s) and their poor, miserable, uncomfortable, *defiling* performance.

And if you are not already impotent, porn very well *will* make you impotent. The need for a stronger fix is a marker along the way to even more impotence.

Stepping back

If "It is all meaningless, it is all meaningless, everything is meaningless," and there are isolated, meaningless pleasures and pains atomized in a meaningless life, then if you're looking for pleasure delivery systems, sex may represent the greatest pleasure that can be used without empty addiction, and for that matter should be used that way, and it is understandable at least to seek what seems like harmless pleasure in porn. The reality of porn addiction may be different. It is, with other evils, a pursuit of something that does not exist and cannot create lasting satisfaction. Not that porn is the only evil by any stretch of the imagination. But it is one way of reaching the misery for which the final destination is a Hell that has many, many entrances but not one exit.

But you are invited to the unsexy (and I am sorry to use the term) advice your parents gave or should have given you, that if the house feels a little cold to you, and you aren't wearing a sweater, put on a sweater. The expedient of lighting part of your house on fire is not a way to stay pleasantly warm; it is an inexpedient that will leave you homeless, and out in the cold.

The words, "Meaningless, meaningless, all is meaningless" open the book of the Bible that poses the terrifying question the rest of the Bible answers.[5] And the Bible, along with the other treasures of the Orthodox Tradition, tell of a world where everything is created with meaning, in which we all of us make an eternal choice between Heaven and Hell, in which the Son of God became a man so that men might become the Sons of God, and in which marriage between one lord and one wife offers the best and most lasting sexual pleasure there is to be had, and which pleasure is transcended as husband and wife grow more and more in love as the years pass and turn into decades. Not, necessarily, that marriage is the only path that can go with salvation: monasticism excels marriage and for that matter married sex. However, marriage is an incredible, wondrous thing, and the sexual aspect of a couple welcoming children (the best sex is when you're trying to make a baby) is part of a wonderful and beautiful picture.

5   Ecclesiastes

Conclusion

G.K. Chesterton wrote in *Orthodoxy: The Romance of Faith* that he set about the business of designing Utopia, and when he had planned a tower, he found it a thousand years old and shining in the sun. He even, he says, thinks he could have invented marriage: he says this somewhat humbly as inventing or even reinventing marriage is an act of creative genius of the first order. Real old-fashioned marriage is an incredible thing. It may be eclipsed in monasticism, and even the place of sexuality in marriage may be eclipsed by the place of sexuality in monasticism. But it is an epic thing, the stuff of which fairy tales and dreams are made of.

Porn is an ever hollow consolation prize next to true marriage. Go for the gold here, not a photoshopped gold-plated turd!

A Pet Owner's Rules

God is a pet owner who has two rules, and only two rules. They are:

1. I am your Owner. Enjoy freely the food and water which I have provided for your good!

2. Don't drink out of the toilet.

That's really it. Those are the only two rules we are expected to follow. And we still break them.

Drunkenness is drinking out of the toilet. If you ask most recovering alcoholics if the time they were drunk all the time were their most joyful, merry, halcyon days, I don't know exactly how they'd answer, if they could even keep a straight face. Far from being joyful, being drunk all the time is misery that most recovering alcoholics wouldn't wish on their worst enemies. If you are drunk all the time, you lose the ability to enjoy much of anything. Strange as it may sound, it takes sobriety to enjoy even drunkenness. Drunkenness is drinking out of the toilet.

Lust is also drinking out of the toilet. Lust is the disenchantment of the entire universe. It is a magic spell where suddenly nothing else is interesting, and after lust destroys the ability to enjoy anything else, lust destroys the ability to enjoy even lust. Proverbs says, "The adulterous woman"—today one might add, "and internet porn" to that —"in the beginning is as sweet as honey and in the end as bitter as gall and as sharp as a double-edged sword." Now this is talking about a lot more than pleasure, but it is talking about pleasure. Lust, a sin of pleasure, ends by destroying pleasure. It takes chastity to enjoy even lust.

Having said that lust is drinking out of the toilet, I'd like to clarify something. There are eight particularly dangerous sins the Church warns us about. That's one, and it isn't the most serious. Sins of lust are among the most easily forgiven; the Church's most scathing condemnations go to sins like pride and running the poverty industry. The harshest condemnations go to sins that are deliberate, cold-blooded sins, not so much disreputable, hot-blooded sins like lust. Lust is drinking out of the toilet, but there are much worse problems.

I'd like you to think about the last time you traveled from one place to another and you enjoyed the scenery. That's good, and it's something that greed destroys. Greed destroys the ability to enjoy things without needing to own them, and there are a lot of things in life (like scenery) that we can enjoy if we are able to enjoy things without always having to make them mine, mine, mine. Greed isn't about enjoying things; it's about grasping and letting the ability to enjoy things slip through your fingers. When people aren't greedy, they know contentment; they can enjoy their own things without wishing they were snazzier or newer or more antique or what have you. (And if you do get that hot possession you've been coveting, greed destroys the ability to simply enjoy it: it becomes as dull and despicable as all your possessions look when you look at them through greed's darkened eyes. It takes contentment to enjoy even greed: greed is *also* drinking out of the toilet.

Jesus had some rather harsh words after being unforgiving after God has forgiven us so much. Even though forgiveness is work, refusing to forgive one other person is drinking out of the toilet. Someone said it's like drinking poison and hoping it will hurt the other person.

The last sin I'll mention is pride, even though all sin is drinking out of the toilet. Pride is not about joy; pride destroys joy. Humility is less about pushing yourself down than an attitude that lets you respect and enjoy others. Pride makes people sneer at others who they can only see as despicable, and when you can't enjoy anyone else, you are too poisoned to enjoy yourself. If you catch yourself enjoying pride, repent of it, but if you can enjoy pride at all, you haven't hit rock bottom. As G.K. Chesterton said, it takes humility to enjoy even pride. Pride is drinking out of the toilet. *All* sin is drinking out of the toilet.

I've talked about drinking out of the toilet, but Rule Number Two is not the focus. Rule Number One is, "I am your owner. Enjoy freely of the food and water I have given you." Rule Number Two, "Don't drink out of the toilet," is only important when we break it, which is unfortunately quite a lot. The second rule is really a footnote meant to help us focus on Rule Number One, the real rule.

What is Rule Number One about? One window that lets us glimpse the beauty of Rule Number One is, "If you have faith the size of a mustard seed, you can say to a mountain, 'Be uprooted and thrown into the sea,' and it will be done for you." Is this exaggeration? Yes. More specifically, it's the kind of exaggeration the Bible uses to emphasize important points. Being human sometimes means that there are mountains that are causing us real trouble. If someone remains in drunkenness and becomes an alcoholic, that alcoholism becomes a mountain that no human strength is strong enough to move. I've known several Christians who were recovering alcoholics. And had been sober for years. *That* is a mountain moved by faith. Without exception, they have become some of the most Christlike, loving people I have known. That is what can happen when we receive freely of the food and drink our Lord provides us. And it's not the only example. There has been an Orthodox resurrection in Albania. Not long ago, it was a church in ruins as part of a country that was ruins. Now the Albanian Orthodox Church is alive and strong, and a powerhouse of transformation for the whole nation. God is on the move in Albania. He's moved mountains.

To eat of the food and drink the Lord has provided—and, leaving the image of dog food behind, this means not only the Eucharist but the whole life God provides—makes us share in the divine nature and live the divine life. We can bring Heaven down to earth, not only beginning ourselves to live the heavenly life, but beginning to establish Heaven around us through our good works. It means that we share in good things we don't always know to ask.

Let's choose the food and drink we were given.

The Magic Stone

There's a picture book by Russel Hoban called *Nothing to Do* that illuminates the value of free time for children, and the importance of helping them learn how to deal with it. Hoban's book opens with little Walter Possum, a member of an endearing family of humanoid possums, who bothers his parents because he has "nothing to do." Father Possum tells Walter to "play with your toys." But Walter doesn't feel like it. The father assigns him a job—to rake the leaves. But Walter soon loses interest. The only activity that seems to relieve the tedium is quarreling with his sister Charlotte, a terrible pest.

When Mother Possum needs to clean the house, Father gives Walter a smooth brown stone and instructs him to run it when he has nothing to do. It is a magic stone, Father tells him. "You have to look around and think while you're rubbing it, and then the stone gives you something to do."

Naturally, belief in the magic of the stone leads Walter to discover all manner of things to do. He finds a long-lost ball, he visits a friend, he dreams up a buried treasure game. He even devises a clever way to keep his irksome little sister from interrupting his game by presenting her with a stick that is also invested with putative magic powers. Besides having fun, he stays out of his parents' hair all afternoon.

Marie Winn, *The Plug-in Drug*

My biggest point taken away from reading *The Plug-in Drug* was that television (today one might add "and Facebook, video games, Facebook games...") drops into the hand as incredibly low-hanging fruit. There are other, more enjoyable and more rewarding things to do with our time (who really feels good after an evening of trawling clickbait?), but they do not do the service of dropping into our hand. This has the result that if you are used to Facebook or TV giving you something to do, it's hard not to sit and do nothing besides staring at the wall because you do not see anything to do.

This article is meant to help you find something to do.

This article, in imitation of a writing prompts page, is intended to remind the reader of other things to do. Many of them are not as easy as Twitter, and some of them involve learning real skill. However, I believe that a good pick from the options here could help us get back from "Nothing to do" besides YouTube.

1. Read *101 Creative Dates: Ideas, Tips, and Personal Experiences from the Life of a Hopeless Romantic* and look for ideas that might apply to you whether or not you have a significant other.

2. Read G.K. Chesterton, *What is Wrong with the World*.

3. Take up adult Legos.

4. Start attending an Orthodox parish.

5. Keep an aquarium.

6. Read and follow up on Sally Fallon, *Nourishing Traditions*, and then Robb Wolf, *The Paleo Solution: The Original Human Diet*.

7. Learn a musical instrument, perhaps a recorder.

8. Learn to sew.

9. Learn the art of memory as in *Kevin Trudeau's Mega Memory* even if it doesn't live up to the advertising hype.

10. Read "Amazing Providence."[6]

11. Learn how to take works from Project Gutenberg and read them in your Kindle or ebook reader. You might start with reading Boethius, *The Consolation of Philosophy*.

12. Take up coin collecting.

13. Take a camping trip.

14. Take up origami.

15. Read " 'Social Antibodies' Needed: A Request of Orthodox Clergy."[7]

16. Take up knitting.

17. Read How Can I Take my Life Back from my Phone?.

18. Read 55 New Maxims for the Cyber-Quarantine.

19. Join a class or activity with your park district.

20. Read "The *Silicon* Rule."[8]

21. Stargaze.

22. Read "The Best Things in Life are Free."[9]

6   cjshayward.com/providence
7   cjshayward.com/social-antibodies
8   cjshayward.com/silicon
9   cjshayward.com/best

23. Take up jewelry making.

24. Read "Ask for the Ancient Ways."[10]

25. Join a book discussion club.

26. Read "The Angelic Letters."[11]

27. Read "Refutatio Omnium Haeresium."[12]

28. Volunteer, perhaps at a local food pantry.

29. Learn to juggle.

30. Explore local tourist attractions.

31. Take up watercolor painting.

32. Read "Beyond the Unbearable Burden of Non-Being."[13]

33. Take up model building.

34. Research and practice active listening.

35. Read "Will There Be a Place for Me?."[14]

---

10 cjshayward.com/ancient
11 cjshayward.com/letters
12 cjshayward.com/refutatio
13 cjshayward.com/beyond
14 cjshayward.com/will-there-be-a-place-for-me

36.Read "What to Own for Happiness (and what not)."[15]

37.Take up amateur acting.

38.Read "Game Review: Meatspace."[16]

39.Buy, and learn to use, a yo-yo. A butterfly yoyo may be easiest.

40.Read "Why I'm Glad I'm Living Now, at This Place, at This Time, in This World."[17]

41.Walk a mile on the sidewalk without stepping on any cracks.

42.Cloudwatch.

43.Go hiking.

44.Read "Yonder."[18]

45.Read "Stephanos."[19]

46.Read "Technology Is Part of Our Poverty."[20]

47.Spend an hour outside.

---

15 cjshayward.com/what-to-own-for-happiness-and-what-not
16 cjshayward.com/meatspace
17 cjshayward.com/why-im-glad-im-alive-now-at-this-time-in-this-world
18 cjshayward.com/yonder
19 cjshayward.com/stephanos
20 cjshayward.com/technology-is-part-of-our-poverty

48. Keep a journal.

49. Read "Plato: The Allegory of the... *Flickering Screen?*"[21]

50. Read "Who is Rich? The Person Who Is Content."[22]

51. Start and keep a blog.

52. Peoplewatch.

53. Read Roger von Oech's *Creative Whack Pack*.

54. Read "Mindfulness and Manners."[23]

55. Take a class at your community college.

56. Read books at *Orthodox Church Fathers*.[24]

57. Read " 'Religion and Science' is not Just Intelligent Design vs. Evolution."[25]

58. Keep a garden.

59. Read Fire in the Hole.

60. Do an act of gratuitous kindness for someone else.

21 cjshayward.com/plato
22 cjshayward.com/contentment-covetousness
23 cjshayward.com/mindfulness-manners
24 orthodoxchurchfathers.com
25 cjshayward.com/religion-science

61. Color an adult coloring book.

62. Write a paper letter to an older relative.

63. Visit a local library and find something to start reading.

64. Read "Revelation and Our Singularity."[26]

65. Learn to be an illusionist for the children in your life.

66. Take up wood burning.

67. Read "Happiness in an Age of Crisis."[27]

68. Read "You Can Choose to be Happy in the Here and Now."[28]

69. Take up a team sport.

70. Take up sudoku.

71. Read "True 'Woke' is Repentance."[29]

72. Take up candle making.

73. Read "How to Find a Job: A Guide for Orthodox Christians."[30]

26 cjshayward.com/revelation-and-our-singularity
27 cjshayward.com/happiness-in-an-age-of-crisis
28 cjshayward.com/you-can-choose-to-be-happy-in-the-here-and-now
29 cjshayward.com/true-woke-repentance
30 cjshayward.com/find-a-job

74. Take up woodworking.

75. Read "Singularity."[31]

76. View and follow up on "Depression is a Disease of Civilization."[32]

77. Keep a pet or, if you cannot responsibly own a pet now, visit at a local pet shelter. You don't need to give the impression that you're looking to adopt; most shelters welcome people who will give the pets constructive attention, and if you ask and a pet shelter says they only want people looking to adopt, say "Thank you," and move on to another one.

78. Read Stephen Covey's *Seven Habits of Highly Effective People.*

79. Dig into the puzzles at *Python Challenge.*[33]

80. Take up oil painting.

81. Read *The Luddite's Guide to Technology.*[34]

82. Do some honest soul-searching, and try to do better.

83. Take up jigsaw puzzles.

---

31 cjshayward.com/singularity
32 tinyurl.com/depression-is-a
33 pythonchallenge.com
34 cjshayward.com/lgt

84. Read "Veni, Vidi, Vomui: A Look at 'Do You Want to Date my Avatar?' "[35]

85. Explore a museum.

86. Read "Physics".[36]

87. Get Lego Mindstorms and start hobbyist robotics.

88. Read "Branding is the New Root of All Evil."[37]

89. Go walking.

90. Take up geocaching.

91. Take up flower arranging.

92. Take up letterboxing.

93. Read "The Consolation of Theology."[38]

94. Give someone a gift.

95. Learn to cook.

96. Volunteer in English as a Second Language instruction.

---

35 cjshayward.com/avatar
36 cjshayward.com/physics
37 cjshayward.com/branding-is-the-new-root-of-all-evil
38 cjshayward.com/consolation

97.Read "Beware of Geeks Bearing Gifts."[39]

98.Learn to play chess.

99.Take up archery.

100.Start birding.

101.Take up bug collecting.

102.Take up sewing.

103.Join Toastmasters.

104.Take up climbing.

105.Apologize to someone you have hurt.

106.Read "A Note to the Reader."[40]

107.Read "Religion Within the Bounds of Amusement."[41]

108.Read "The Arena."[42]

109.Take up stamp collecting.

110.Ask to join a group of people playing sports or talking in the park.

39 cjshayward.com/geeks
40 cjshayward.com/reader
41 cjshayward.com/amusement
42 cjshayward.com/arena

111. Take up crossword puzzles.

112. Become a clown.

113. Take up balloon sculpting and make balloons for the children you know.

Enjoy any one of these, or just a few.

Fire in the Hole

The professor continued his reading.

> In *The Divine Names* I have shown the sense
> in which God is described as good, existent,
> life, wisdom, power, and whatever other
> things pertain to the conceptual names for
> God. In my *Symbolic Theology* I have
> discussed analogies of God drawn from what
> we perceive. I have spoken of the images we
> have of him, of the forms, figures, and
> instruments proper to him, of the places in
> which he lives and the ornaments which he
> wears. I have spoken of his anger, grief, and
> rage, of how he is said to be drunk and
> hungover, of his oaths and curses, of his
> sleeping and waking, and indeed of all those
> images we have of him, images shaped by the

workings of the representations of God. And I
feel sure that you have noticed how these
latter come much more abundantly than what
went before, since *The Theological
Representations* and a discussion of the
names appropriate to God are inevitably
briefer than what can be said in *The Symbolic
Theology*. The fact is that the more we take
flight upward, the more find ourselves not
simply running short of words but actually
speechless and unknowing. In the earlier
books my argument this downward path from
the most exalted to the humblest categories,
taking in on this downward path an ever-
increasing number of ideas which multiplied
what is below up to the transcendent, and the
more it climbs, the more language falters, and
when it has passed up and beyond the ascent,
it will turn silent completely, since it will
finally be at one with him who is
indescribable.

Now you may wonder why it is that, after
starting out from the highest category when
our method involves assertions, we begin now
from the lowest category involves a denial.
The reason is this. When we assert what is
beyond every assertion, we must then proceed
from what is most akin to it, and as we do so
we make the affirmation on which everything
else depends. But when we deny that which is
beyond every denial, we have to start by

denying those qualities which differ most from the goal we hope to attain. Is it not closer to truth to say that God is life and goodness rather than that he is air or stone? Is it not more accurate to deny that drunkenness and rage can be attributed to him than to deny that we can apply to him the terms of speech and thought?

So this is what we say. The Cause of all is above all and is not inexistent, lifeless, speechless, mindless. It is not a material body, and hence has neither shape nor form, quality, quantity, or weight. It is not in any place and can be neither seen nor touched. It is neither perceived nor is it perceptible. It suffers neither disorder nor disturbance and is overwhelmed by no earthly passion. It is not powerless and subject to the disturbances caused by sense perception. It endures no deprivation of light. It passes through no change, decay, division, loss, no ebb and flow, nothing of which the senses may be aware. None of this can either be identified with it nor attributed.

Again, as we climb higher we say this. It is not soul or mind, nor does it possess imagination, conviction, speech, or understanding. Nor is it speech per se, understanding per se. It cannot be spoken of and it cannot be grasped by understanding. It is not number or order, greatness or smallness, equality or inequality, similarity or dissimilarity. It is not immovable, moving, or at rest. It has no power, it is not power, nor is it light. It does not live nor is it light. It does not live nor is it life. It is not a substance, nor is it eternity or time. It cannot be grasped by the understanding since it is neither knowledge nor truth. It is not kingship. It is not wisdom. It is neither one nor oneness, divinity nor goodness. Nor is it a spirit, in the sense in which we understand the term. It is not sonship or fatherhood and it is nothing known to us or any other being. Existing beings do not know it as it actually is and it does not know them as they are. There is no speaking of it, nor name or knowledge of it. Darkness and light, error and truth—it is none of these. It is beyond assertion and denial. We make assertions and denials of what is next to it, but never of it, for it is both beyond every assertion, being the perfect and unique cause of all things, and, by virtue of its preeminently simple and absolute nature, free of every limitation, beyond every limitation, it is also beyond every denial.

Prof. Sarovsky slowly and reverently closed the book. "St. Dionysius says elsewhere that God is known by every name and no name, and that everything that is is a name of God. And in fact in discussing symbols which have some truth but are necessarily inadequate to reality, crude symbols are to be preferred to those which appear elevated, since even their 'crassness' is a 'goad' spurring us to reach higher."

"So now I'd like to have an exercise. Could somebody please name something at random, and I can tell how it tells the glory of God?"

A young man from the back called out, "Porn."

Prof. Sarovsky said, "Ha ha, hysterical. Could I have another suggestion?"

Another young man called out, "Porn."

Prof. Sarovsky said, "I'm serious. Porn, when you start using it, seems to be a unique spice. But the more you use it, the more it actually *drains* spice from everything else, and eventually drains itself, and when pornography can only go so far, you find yourself not only jailed but charged with rape. Lustfulness is in the beginning as sweet as honey and in the end as bitter as gall and as sharp as a double-edged sword. And much as I disagree with feminists on important points, I agree with a feminist dictionary: 'Pornography is the theory; rape is the practice.' Could I have a serious suggestion?"

A couple of cellphones started playing, "Internet is for porn."

Prof. Sarovsky called on the class's most vocal feminist. "Delilah! Would you pick a topic?"

Delilah grinned wickedly and said, "I'm with the boys on this one. Porn."

Prof. Sarovsky paused briefly and says, "Very well, then, porn it is. The famous essay 'I, Pencil' takes the humble pencil up and just starts to dig and dig at the economic family tree of just what resources and endeavors make up the humble lead pencil. So it talks about logging, and all the work in transporting the wood, and the mining involved in the graphite, and the exquisite resources that go just to make the blue strip on the metal band, and so on and so forth, and the 'rubber' eraser and whatnot. The conclusion is that millions of dollars' resources (he does not calculate a figure) went into making a humble wooden pencil, and he pushes further: only God knows how to make a pencil. And if only God knows how to make a pencil, a fortiori only God knows how to make a porn site...

"And, I suppose, a pencil must be a phallic symbol."

Then he paused, and said, "Just kidding!"

The room was silent.

Prof. Sarovsky bowed deeply and grinned: "I'll see you and raise you."

And this is what he said.

I, Porn, want to tell you about myself. There are options that eclipse me, but I can make my point more strongly if I speak for myself, Porn, who represent myriads of wonders.

It is not my point in particular that only God knows how to make a Porn site. The point has been well enough made that only God knows how to make a pencil, and is a less interesting adjustment to acknowledge that only God knows how to make a Porn site.

Nor do I suggest that the straight-laced print off a Porn image and frame and hang it on the wall. Though if they understood my lineage, the question would then become whether they were worthy to do so.

I have a magnificent and vaster lineage than "I, Pencil" begins to draw out. A brilliance in economics, the author simply underscores a great interdependent web of economic resources in the humble pencil's family tree.

Equipment, mining, logging, transportation: the economic underpinnings of a humble pencil amount to millions of dollars, and the details mentioned only scratch the surface even of the economics involved.

I have a vaster lineage, including such things as war in Heaven. Now the war in Heaven is over, and was over when the Archangel Michael only said his name, which in the Hebrew tongue says, "Who is like God?" and with that, the devils were cast down, sore losers afflicting the Royal Race one and all. And even then, it was only angelic spirits that could come anywhere close to their war against God. Even then, they are limited. They are on a leash. Perhaps someday I will tell you of why you are summoned to a holy and blinding arrogance towards that whole camp.

What is the Royal Race? I get ahead of myself.

I, Porn, don't merely share a universe with the divine virtues. In my production there is the cutting off of self-will, long suffering, and as little lust as might be found in a monastery. Dostoevsky offers the image of the chaste harlot; I can add only that if Christ were walking today, Porn models would be among the first he would associate with.

The core impulse I, Porn, draw on, is good. It is a testament to the human spirit that nine months after a natural disaster, there is a wave of babies born. The core impulse is the impulse for the preservation of the species, the possibility by which a community of mortals has itself no automatic end.

It is closer to my point to say that God is not just good and divine; he has created a world that in every way reflects his grandeur. There are no small parts: only actors who are not really small. Every superstring vibration in the cosmos is grander and vaster than all the pagan gods of all worlds put together.

Or as G.K. Chesterton said, "Once I planned to write a book of poems entirely about the things in my pocket. But I found it would be too long; and the age of the great epics is past."

It is still closer to my majesty to observe Alexander Solzhenitsyn, who suffered in the Gulag that Hitler sent observers for inspiration for Nazi concentration camps, "Gradually it was disclosed to me that the line separating good and evil passes not through states, nor between classes, not between political parties either — but right through every heart — and through all human hearts. This line shifts. Inside us, it oscillates with the years. And even within hearts overwhelmed by evil, one small bridgehead of good is retained. And even in the best of all hearts, there remains . . . an unuprooted small corner of evil."

The Heavens declare the glory of God—and so do I, Porn.

Perhaps the most beautiful doctrine in Origen that Orthodox must condemn is the final and ultimate salvation of all Creation: that the Devil himself will be a last prodigal son returning to home in Heaven. But the Orthodox teaching is more beautiful: a teaching that every spiritual being, every man, every fallen or unfallen angel, is given an eternal choice between Heaven and Hell and not one of these will God rape, however much he desires their salvation. To quote The Dark Tower: "A man can't be taken to hell, or sent to hell: you can only get there on your own steam." God has made a rock he could not could move, and that rock is man and angel.

The rising crescendo that practically seals C.S. Lewis, "The Weight of Glory," is:

> It is a serious thing to live in a society of possible gods and goddesses, to remember that the dullest and most uninteresting person you talk to may one day be a creature which, if you saw it now, you would be strongly tempted to worship, or else a horror and a corruption such as you now meet, if at all, only in a nightmare. All day long we are, in some degree, helping each other to one or other of these destinations. It is in the light of these overwhelming possibilities, it is with the awe and the circumspection proper to them, that we should conduct all our dealings with one another, all friendships, all loves, all play, all politics. There are no ordinary people. You have never talked to a mere mortal. Nations, cultures, arts, civilization—these are mortal, and their life is to ours as the life of a gnat. But it is immortals whom we joke with, work with, marry, snub, and exploit—immortal horrors or everlasting splendours.

Which brings us to the messy circumstances of your lives.

George Bernard Shaw said, "There are two tragedies in life. One is not to get your heart's desire. The other is to get it." We can see it, perhaps in a fantasy setting, in a passage from C.S. Lewis, *The Voyage of the Dawn Treader*, has Lucy tiptoe to a room with a spellbook and see a singular spell:

(Read this copyrighted passage at tinyurl.com/lucys-spell.)

The temptation, patterned after real temptation of the real world, is to want a horror. It is because Lucy is bewitched that she even wants what the spell promises. The destruction of kingdoms when lords vie for her beauty? Women may want to feel like the most beautiful woman in the world, but the count in stacking dead bodies like cordwood is no true metric for beauty. As a faithfully portrayed temptation by C.S. Lewis, what is being desired is not something Heavenly. It is a vision of Hell, pure and simple. While in the grips of temptation, she could not be happy without casting that spell until she let go of it from a strong warning from Aslan. But even if she succeeded, she would be even more unhappy. Her success would rival world wars or nuclear wars in its destruction of beautiful worlds, and if it didn't bring her death, she would live on in a wrecked world, knowing for the rest of her life that it was her petty self-absorption that obliterated the majesty of worlds.

Even if we scale from back from undisguised fantasy, we can look at what is a practical possibility for some people in the real world. Cameron Russell's "Looks Aren't Everything. Believe me, I'm a model." The TED talk eloquently explains that being a supermodel is not all sunshine and not the solution to all life's problems. For that matter it isn't even the solution to *body image* problems, and the final point she shares is that as a model she has to be *more*, not less, insecure about her body, no matter how lovely she may appear to others. It turns out that supermodels are intimidated by... other supermodels. Being a model is not a way to be exempt from body image struggles.

And this is in no way a solely a phenomenon about body image. There is one man where professional opinion is that he is smarter than most genuises, and that the average Harvard PhD has never met someone so talented. And his work history, given that he's tried to give his best? Here's something really odd. One job assistant said, "You don't want your boss figuring out you're smarter than him." When he hands in his first piece of work, only some bosses respond kindly to work that is beyond the boss's wildest dreams. Most of them find themselves in unfamiliar social territory, and strike out or retaliate. He's been terminated a dozen times and is now retired on disability, the best financial arrangement he has had yet. It may be true, up to a point, that there's something likable about being smart. That doesn't mean in any sense that the smarter you get, the more people like you, or that your life is easy.

There is a portal that far excels entering another world, entering Narnia, Hogwarts, or Middle Earth. And this portal is much harder to see or look for than Narnia. It is entering the here and now you have been placing.

Spiritual masters have said to want what you have, not what you don't have, and want things to be for you just the way they are. Now there is such a thing as legitimately seeking to solve, lessen, or improve a problem, and wishing you had a better-paying job, a car, or a nicer house. Wishing never runs out, and if you get the Apple Watch you want, wishing will just wish for newer or different things. Buy something you don't need but will make you enchanted for a month. *I dare you.*

Oh, and by the way, I, Porn, know all about wishing. I know *everything* about it, and I know everything it *can't* do.

When you let go of escape, soon you may let go of relating the here and now as the sort of thing one should flee, and some thick, sticky grey film will slowly melt away from your eyes and they will open on beauty all around you, and you will have crossed a threshold no fantasy portal even comes close. And you will have every treasure that you have. And perhaps, in and through ancient religion or postmodern positive psychology, cultivate a deep and abiding gratefulness for all the blessings you have.

In the Way of Things, there are two basic options one can pursue. One is the Sexual Way, and the other is the Hyper-Sexual Way. Let me explain.

Study after study has been launched to investigate which group of mavericks has the best sex, and they have been repeatedly been dismayed to find that the overlooked Sexual Way has the most pleasure. The overlooked Sexual Way is that of a contest of love, for life, between one lord and one wife, chaste before the wedding and faithful after, grateful for children, and knowing that the best sex ever is when you are trying to make a baby. After the first year or two some outward signs get quiet and subdued, but the marriage succeeds because the honeymoon has failed. It deepens year after year and decade after a decade, and a widowed senior can say, "You don't know what love is when you're a kid." And here, like no other place, beauty is forged in the eye of the beholder. Here, unlike fashion magazines, sweaty fitness regimens, and dieting, and weighing, and accursed "bodysculpting," a woman can and should be made to feel like she is the most beautiful woman in the world, to a husband to whom she really is the most beautiful woman in the world, as naturally as the Church on Sunday. As Homer and Marge humbly and quietly sing to each other, "You are so *beautiful* to me!"

If the sexual impulse is spent wisely in the Sexual Way, it is invested at exorbitant interest on the Hyper-Sexual Way. Wonder what all that curious monastic modesty about? It compounds an essential sexual condition, by which a monastic, man or woman, becomes a transgendered god and his sexual desire is entirely fixed on God. Does this seem strange? Let us listen to St. Herman of Alaska:

> Further on Yanovsky writes, "Once the Elder was invited aboard a frigate which came from Saint Petersburg. The Captain of the frigate was a highly educated man, who had been sent to America by order of the Emperor to make an inspection of all the colonies. There were more than twenty-five officers with the Captain, and they also were educated men. In the company of this group sat a monk of a hermitage, small in stature and wearing very old clothes. All these educated conversationalists were placed in such a position by his wise talks that they did not know how to answer him. The Captain himself used to say, 'We were lost for an answer before him.'

> "Father Herman gave them all one general question: 'Gentlemen, What do you love above all, and what will each of you wish for your

happiness?' Various answers were offered ...
Some desired wealth, others glory, some a
beautiful wife, and still others a beautiful ship
he would captain; and so forth in the same
vein. 'It is not true,' Father Herman said to
them concerning this, 'that all your various
wishes can bring us to one conclusion—that
each of you desires that which in his own
understanding he considers the best, and
which is most worthy of his love?' They all
answered, 'Yes, that is so!' He then continued,
'Would you not say, Is not that which is best,
above all, and surpassing all, and that which
by preference is most worthy of love, the Very
Lord, our Jesus Christ, who created us,
adorned us with such ideals, gave life to all,
sustains everything, nurtures and loves all,
who is Himself Love and most beautiful of all
men? Should we not then love God above
every thing, desire Him more than anything,
and search Him out?'

"All said, 'Why, yes! That's self-evident!' Then
the Elder asked, 'But do you love God?' They
all answered, 'Certainly, we love God. How can
we not love God?' 'And I a sinner have been
trying for more than forty years to love God, I
cannot say that I love Him completely,' Father
Herman protested to them. He then began to
demonstrate to them the way in which we
should love God. 'If we love someone,' he said,
'we always remember them; we try to please

them. Day and night our heart is concerned with the subject. Is that the way you gentlemen love God? Do you turn to Him often? Do you always remember Him? Do you always pray to Him and fulfill His holy commandments?' They had to admit that they had not! 'For our own good, and for our own fortune,' concluded the Elder, 'let us at least promise ourselves that from this very minute we will try to love God more than anything and to fulfill His Holy Will!' Without any doubt this conversation was imprinted in the hearts of the listeners for the rest of their lives.'

Fr. Herman had something better than pixels on a screen. **Much** better.

Perhaps the most controversial argument in the history of philosophy is by Anselm of Canterbury, who said, "If God exists, nothing greater than him could exist. Now God either exists in reality and also in our minds, or only as a concept in our minds. But to exist in reality as well as our minds is greater than to exist only in our minds. Therefore, God must have the higher excellence of existing in reality as well as our minds."

I am not specifically interested in bringing agreement or disagreement to this argument. First, most people first meeting this argument feel that something has been slipped past them, but they can't put a finger on where the error is. However, I did not exactly include this argument to discuss what it *asserts*, but what it *assumes*: if God is greater than anything else that can be thought, then we have something that pierces deeply into the Christian God.

The joke is told that four rabbis would get together to discuss Torah, and one specific rabbi was the odd man out, every single time. And they said, "Three against one." Finally, the exasperated odd rabbi out knelt down, prayed, "Gd, I've worked very hard, and they never listen. Please send them a sign that I'm right." It was a warm day out, but a sudden chilly wind blew by, and some clouds appeared in the sky. The other three rabbis said, "That's odd, but it's still three against one." Then the rabbi knelt down, prayed, "Please make a clearer sign," and the wind grew more bitter and it began sleeting. The rabbi said, "Well?" The other rabbis said, "This is quite a coincidence, but it's still three against one." Then before the rabbi could begin to pray, bolts of lightning splintered a nearby tree, there was an earthquake, the earth opened, and a deep voice thundered, "HE'S RIGHT!" The rabbi said, "Well?" Quick as a flash, another rabbi said, "*Well?* It's still three against two!"

The humor element in this element extends beyond, "If God has spoken, the discussion is over." The humor element hinges on the fact that counting does not go from "one, two, three, four" to "one, two, three, four, *Five*": there is infinite confusion in adding one God to four men. As written in "Doxology:"[43]

> Thou who art One,
> Eternally beyond time,
> So wholly One,
> That thou mayest be called infinite,
> Timeless beyond time thou art,

43 cjshayward.com/doxology

The One who is greater than infinity art thou.
Father, Son, and Holy Spirit,
The Three who are One,
No more bound by numbers than by word,
And yet the Son is called Ο ΛΟΓΟΣ,
The Word,
Divine ordering Reason,
Eternal Light and Cosmic Word,
Way pre-eminent of all things,
Beyond all, and infinitesimally close,
Thou transcendest transcendence itself,
The Creator entered into his Creation,
Sharing with us humble glory,
Lowered by love,
Raised to the highest,
The Suffering Servant known,
The King of Glory,
Ο ΩΝ....

Wert thou a lesser god,
Numerically one as a creature is one,
Only one by an accident,
Naught more,
Then thou couldst not deify thine own
creation,
Whilst remaining the only one god.

But thou art beyond all thought,
All word, all being,
We may say that thou existest,
But then we must say,
Thou art, I am not.

And if we say that we exist,
It is inadequate to say that thou existest,
For thou art the source of all being,
And beyond our being;
Thou art the source of all mind, wisdom, and
reason,
Yet it is a fundamental error to imagine thee,
To think and reason in the mode of mankind.
Thou art not one god because there happeneth
not more,
Thou art The One God because there mighteth
not be another beside thee.
Thus thou spakest to Moses,
Thou shalt have no other gods before me.
Which is to say,
Thou shalt admit no other gods to my
presence.

And there can be no other god beside thee,
So deep and full is this truth,
That thy Trinity mighteth take naught from
thine Oneness,
Nor could it be another alongside thy divine
Oneness,
If this God became man,
That man become god.

The Trinity does not represent a weaker or less
consistent monotheism than Islam. The Trinity represents a
stronger and more consistent monotheism than Islam, and
that is why it can afford things that are unthinkable to a
Muslim.

A Hindu once asked a Christian, "I can accept the truth of the incarnation, but why only one?" And in that conversation, where the Christian defended only one incarnation, both were wrong. Or rather, the Christian was wrong; the Hindu was merely mistaken.

Q. 1. What is the chief end of man?

A. Man's chief end is to glorify God, and to BECOME him forever.

One theology professor tried to explain to a Muslim that the Trinity is how Christians get to the absolute Oneness of God. The men who first articulated the doctrine looked with some horror on the concept of using the word "Trinity" as a handle for the doctrine.

Regarding the Hindu mentioned, I would say that there have been many, many true incarnations of God, and they still continue. Now the Hindu concept of an Avatar can be what Christianity rejected as docetistic, with Christ not recognized to have real flesh. However, what I would rather have been said is this: No one besides Christ enters the world with part or all of God as part of them. However, the reason for the coming of the Son of God is to destroy the devil's work. An ancient hymn states, "Trying to be god, Adam failed to be God. Christ became man, to make Adam god." And the vast company of Saints that God keeps on giving are in fact the gift of a company of Avatars; we just have a different understanding of how one reaches a very similar goal.

The *Philokalia* says, "Blessed is the monk who regards each man as God after God."

St. John Chrysostom comments on the Scripture: "We beheld," he says, "His glory, the glory as of the Only-Begotten of the Father."

Having declared that we were made "sons of God," and having shown in what manner5 namely, by the "Word" having been "made Flesh," he again mentions another advantage which we gain from this same circumstance. What is it? "We beheld His glory, the glory as of the Only-Begotten of the Father"; which we could not have beheld, had it not been shown to us, by means of a body like to our own. For if the men of old time could not even bear to look upon the glorified countenance of Moses, who partook of the same nature with us, if that just man needed a veil which might shade over the purity7 of his glory, and show to them have face of their prophet mild and gentle; how could we creatures of clay and earth have endured the unveiled Godhead, which is unapproachable even by the powers above? Wherefore He tabernacled among us, that we might be able with much fearlessness to approach Him, speak to, and converse with Him.

But what means "the glory as of the Only-Begotten of the Father"? Since many of the Prophets too were glorified, as this Moses himself, Elijah, and Elisha, the one encircled by the fiery chariot (2 Kings vi. 17), the other

taken up by it; and after them, Daniel and the
Three Children, and the many others who
showed forth wonders; and angels who have
appeared among men, and partly disclosed to
beholders the flashing light of their proper
nature; and since not angels only, but even the
Cherubim were seen by the Prophet in great
glory, and the Seraphim also: the Evangelist
leading us away from all these, and removing
our thoughts from created things, and from
the brightness of our fellow-servants, sets us
at the very summit of good. For, "not of
prophet," says he, "nor angel, nor archangel,
nor of the higher power, nor of any other
created nature," if other there be, but of the
Master Himself, the King Himself, the true
Only-Begotten Son Himself, of the Very Lord
of all, did we "behold the glory."

For the expression "as," does not in this place
belong to similarity or comparison, but to
confirmation and unquestionable definition;
as though he said, "We beheld glory, such as it
was becoming, and likely that He should
possess, who is the Only-Begotten and true
Son of God, the King of all." The habit (of so
speaking) is general, for I shall not refuse to
strengthen my argument even from common
custom, since it is not now my object to speak
with any reference to beauty of words, or
elegance of composition, but only for your
advantage; and therefore there is nothing to

prevent my establishing my argument by the
instance of a common practice. What then is
the habit of most persons? Often when any
have seen a king richly decked, and glittering
on all sides with precious stones, and are
afterwards describing to others the beauty, the
ornaments, the splendor, they enumerate as
much as they can, the glowing tint of the
purple robe, the size of the jewels, the
whiteness of the mules, the gold about the
yoke, the soft and shining couch. But when
after enumerating these things, and other
things besides these, they cannot, say what
they will, give a full idea of the splendor, they
immediately bring in: "But why say much
about it; once for all, he was like a king;" not
desiring by the expression "like," to show that
he, of whom they say this, resembles a king,
but that he is a real king. Just so now the
Evangelist has put the word As, desiring to
represent the transcendent nature and
incomparable excellence of His glory.

Elsewhere we are asked to consider what things
would be like if a King were to take up residence in one of
the houses of a city. Would not the entire city, and each
house in it, be forever honored? And the Son of God is now
one of our homeboys. He ascended into Heaven and
brought us with him, enthroned in Heaven with him.

We are the Royal Race. We are made in the image of
God, and made to reach unimaginable glory.

And there may be named three laws that are the Constitution of the Royal Race, three laws which are one and the same.

The first law is the Law of the Canoe, as C.S. Lewis summarized his friend Charles Williams:

> It is Virgil himself who died without reaching the *patria*, who saw 'Italy' only from a wave before he was engulfed forever. It is Virgil himself who stretches out his hands among the ghosts *ripae ulterioris amore*, longing to pass a river that he cannot pass. This poet from whose work so many Christians have drawn spiritual nourishment was not himself a Christian—did not himself know the full meaning of his own poetry, for (in Keble's fine words) 'thoughts beyond their thought to those high bards were given'. This is exquisite cruelty; he made honey not for himself; he helped to save others, himself he could not save.

> ...The Atonement was a Substitution, just as Anselm said. But that Substitution, far from being a mere legal fiction irrelevant to the normal workings of the universe, was simply the supreme instance of a universal law. 'He saved others, himself he cannot save' is a *definition* of the Kingdom. All salvation, everywhere and at all times, in great things or in little, is vicarious. The courtesy of the Emperor has absolutely decreed that no man can paddle his own canoe and every man can

paddle his fellow's, so that the shy offering and modest acceptance of indispensable aid shall be the very form of the celestial etiquette. [emphasis original]

The second law is the Law of the Long Spoon. As one telling goes from a liberal enough source:

One day a man said to God, "God, I would like to know what Heaven and Hell are like."

God showed the man two doors. Inside the first one, in the middle of the room, was a large round table with a large pot of stew. It smelled delicious and made the man's mouth water, but the people sitting around the table were thin and sickly. They appeared to be famished. They were holding spoons with very long handles and each found it possible to reach into the pot of stew and take a spoonful, but because the handle was longer than their arms, they could not get the spoons back into their mouths.

The man shuddered at the sight of their misery and suffering. God said, "You have seen Hell."

Behind the second door, the room appeared exactly the same. There was the large round table with the large pot of wonderful stew that made the man's mouth water. The people had the same long-handled spoons, but they were well nourished and plump, laughing and talking.

The man said, "I don't understand."

God smiled. "It is simple," he said, "These people share and feed one another. While the greedy only think of themselves..."

The last law is the Law of Narcissus's Mirror. It states that the Royal Race are absolutely *forbidden* to stand and gaze at themselves in Narcissus's Mirror, entranced at their own beauty, and *commanded* to gaze at other members of the Royal Race, entranced at *their* beauty.

These three laws are one and the same. One joke, about "communio" theologians who hold the Trinity to mean that God himself is a community, ran:

Q: How many communio theologians does it take to change a light bulb?

A: Only one, but he thinks he is a community.

But we are *not* communities. We are *part* of a community, and the full grandeur of being a member of the Royal Race is that you are no *island*, but a connected and beautiful part of a *continent*.

And furthermore, God has ordered Heaven and Earth for the benefit of us as the Royal Race.

Though this may be more subtle in the Sexual Way than in the Hyper-Sexual Way, but the behavior enjoined on the Hyper-Sexual Way is that of a spiritual miser, who constantly thinks his Heavenly wealth is too little and he must spare no effort to get more, and no matter how much treasure in Heaven he acquires, he never rests on his laurels, but keeps on storing up more and more and more.

Men each have one interest, one *real* interest, and only *one* interest: a good answer before the Dread Judgment-Throne of Christ. This life is inestimably precious, and in treasures such as repentance, Heaven's best-kept secret,[44] we can only store up these treasures before this fleeting life is over. Now the Church Triumphant is no terrible place to be, but there are profound goods that are only open to us, the living, for as long as we live. And the various strange prescriptions of the Philokalia and the Orthodox Way, about believing oneself to be the worst of sinners, about giving oneself no credit for any good actions, about believing "All the world will be saved and I will be damned," about repenting as if one will die tomorrow but treating your body as if it will last for many years, are in fact braces to support being one hoarding spiritual miser for the rest of one's life, and crossing the finish line, in triumph, and with treasure after treasure after treasure in your hoard. It is explained that God conceals from us the day of our death, because if we knew we would not die for some decades, we would put off repentance and be incorrigible. Not that God is absolutely unwilling to reveal to people the day of their death: it is in fact considered a mark of holiness to know that, because a person is in a good enough state for the secret not to need to be hidden. But the Philokalia's discussion, perhaps here most clearly of all, explains that things are ordered this way because God has stacked the deck, in *our* favor. And as regards the Sexual Way, the path

44 cjshayward.com/repentance

is said not to be an environment for children to grow up, but an environment for parents to grow up.

And God's Providence is not just Providence in great things. It is Providence in the small. It is not just Providence in a career, or entering the Sexual Way. It is also Providence when you are stuck in traffic and the light seems never to be turning green and that still, small voice urges you to grow just a little as a person so you can be as happy in your car as in a lounge chair at home. And it is the mighty arm of Providence all the more powerfully revealed when we are persecuted, or lose money, or any number of other things. And it is a Providence that gives you the here and now, a here and now chosen for you from all eternity, and will, if you cooperate, help you appreciate the gift.

And if you are one of the many who believe that I, Porn, am the only interesting spice in a fatally dull world, I, Porn, can only say this:

Watch me when I am Transfigured.

To quote your own age's little reflection of The Divine Comedy:

(Read this online at tinyurl.com/oily-ghost.)

An Orthodox would realize in the Burning Angel a clearest reference to the fiery Seraphim, the highest of the nine angel choirs, and the one for whom St. Seraphim of Sarov came, the most beloved Orthodox saint in centuries, the St. Seraphim whose extraordinary conversation with the pilgrim Motovilov[45] reveals the purpose of human life.

We live in interesting times. There is a singularity, or rather has been but keeps growing exponentially, and this singularity may turn in to the end of the world: a strange Ragnarok where the forces of Good resound with

45 http://orthochristian.com/47866.html

apocalyptic triumph. And I, Porn, am part of the singularity, an important part.

Did you know that I, Porn, am not the only thing in life?

Remember: *"Every man who visits a Porn site is looking for God."*

Delilah friend turned back. "Yep, dear, he does that sort of thing in practically every class."

Conclusion

An apocryphal story tells of a Greek philosopher who was approached by a man who said he wanted Truth. The philosopher and presently the man approaching him were both standing in a river.

The philosopher asked the man, "What do you want?"

The man said, "Truth!"

The philosopher pushed the man below the current for a moment and then brought him up asking, "What do you want?"

The man said, "Truth!"

The philosopher pushed the man back down and held him under the water a little longer before bringing him up, and asked, "What do you want?"

The man said, "Truth!"

The philosopher then pushed him down a third time, and continued to hold him under when the man struggled to get away from his grip, and continued still longer until the man had passed out, then let him up and asked, "What do you want?"

The man gasped, "**AIR!**"

The philosopher said, "When you want Truth the way you want air, then you will find it!"

The same principle applies to freedom from porn and freedom from masturbation.

I would briefly pause to note that the Philokalia says, "That which is not desired is of short duration." When I implicitly pray, "Lord, give me chastity, but not quite yet," by fighting and praying against lewd thoughts but wanting to be in the mental images right now, the temptation is long-lasting and it has crossed the line from temptation into sin. When I genuinely do not want a sexual temptation, it is short-lived.

But let us go to slash-and-burn wanting purity like we want air.

The Sermon on the Mount says that if your eye causes you to sin, gouge it out and cast it away, and this is an exaggeration. Subsequent tradition has made it clear that bodily mutilation is not ever the right way to resist sin. But there is something to be said for wanting chastity the way you want air, and destroying anything that gets in your way.

What, for instance, if your new iPhone is a source of sin and addiction, and possibly not just in porn, you drive over it with your car and purchase a talk + text + GPS—*and no porn*—flip-phone from SunbeamWireless.com? I might delicately suggest that that is a lot easier than a divorce. *A piece of cake!*

What about, on a more modest scale, lending your computer to a friend for safekeeping and only checking email from libraries and public computers?

There are a number of steps you can take, and some of them involve getting away from some things for a little while, making them temporarily unavailable while you work on getting grounded. Once you have reached the point of going as slash and burn as you have to, patterns of possibility for purity open up.

And if you care about the broader picture of addictive technology (is your iPhone terrible for productivity even on a work network where most porn sites are blocked?), dig into *Hidden Price Tags: An Eastern Orthodox Look at the Dark Side of Technology and Its Best Use*.[46] It may be the next step to taking control once you have unplugged seductively easy access to porn.

Think about it.

46 cjshayward.com/hpt

9 798869 394866